GW00602612

KNOW YOUR

NEW ZEALAND

BIRDS

by Murdoch Riley

NATIVE LAND BIRDS
Page 3

INTRODUCED LAND BIRDS
Page 43

SEA BIRDS
Page 57

Illustrations by P.F. Scaife

© VIKING SEVENSEAS NZ LTD;
P.O. Box 152, Paraparaumu
Ninth Printing 2005

Because New Zealand has been isolated by sea from other land masses for about seventy million years, its native bird life includes species that have few or no relatives in the world today. The ancestors of flightless birds like the kiwi and takahe must have reached the country when a land bridge existed and are unique. In the absence of any mammalian predators (the tuatara, a few lizards, three species of frogs, and two species of bat were the only native animals) a special evolutionary pattern was able to develop which produced, out of approximately two hundred and fifty species native to New Zealand, many varieties found nowhere else.

The proximity of Australia and the prevailing westerly winds account from the Australian origin of many of our birds. Some, like the pied stilt, came before European settlement, whilst others, such as the Australian coot, are newcomers. The clearing of native vegetation meant the extinction, or near-extinction, of a number of species adapted to forest life. Others coped with introduced predators and to the changes in the enviroment. Through the active conservation efforts of bodies such as the Wildlife Service and Department of Conservation, much progress has been made in preserving rare species of land and sea birds and most are now holding their own.

The aim of this booklet is to provide ready information and illustrations of New Zealand's most commonly seen birds. With one or two exceptions, rare species of birds, such as those surviving only on outlying islands or remote wilderness areas, have been omitted. Sixty seven species have been described, of a known number of now nearly three hundred. Native land birds included number forty and are described in Part One, seventeen introduced land birds in Part Two and eleven sea birds in Part Three. Classification of species in each section follows that of the Annotated Checklist of New Zealand Birds (Reeds), starting with the earliest arrivals.

Front Cover: Kea — see p. 25

The publishers wish to thank the Wildlife Service and Department of Conservation for the loan of some of the bird illustrations, the use of some text from "Forest Wildlife" and their general assistance in compilation of this booklet.

    ISBN 085467 067X

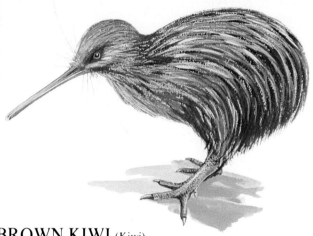

BROWN KIWI (Kiwi)
Apteryx australis

Size:	46 - 56cm.
Status:	Fairly common.
Range:	Throughout the North Island but rarely reported south of the Manawatu Gorge. Northern and western parts of the South Island, Stewart Island.
Habitat:	Native forests, forest remnants and scrub-land.
Description:	Overall greyish brown but with much variation in plumage. Upper parts are sometimes streaked with black, under parts pale grey-brown. Rudimentary wings are hidden in plumage.
Food:	Insects and worms, often obtained by probing in ground; and forest fruits.
Voice:	Male a shrill, repeated, drawn out whistle "Kiwi", female a hoarse cry.
Breeding:	July-February. One to two white eggs which are remarkably large compared to the size of the bird.
General:	North Island, South Island and Stewart Island birds are considered to be of separate subspecies. The differences, however, are not readily apparent in the field. A nocturnal bird found mostly in forest areas. The female is bigger than the male, the size of a domestic hen. Fully protected.

BLACK SHAG (Kawau) (Common Cormorant)
Phalacrocorax carbo

Size:	88cm.
Status:	Common.
Range:	Throughout main islands and some off-shore islands, including Chatham Island.
Habitat:	Inland waters, rivers and sea coast
Description:	Black with greenish tinge both on head and under parts. White patches at throat and on thighs in breeding months. Legs and feet black.
Food:	Trout, eels, all fresh water fish, but not exclusively.
Voice:	Harsh croak and whistle.
Breeding:	October-May. Three to four blue-green eggs.
General:	The largest shag represented in New Zealand. It swims and dives well, but has an ungainly waddle on land. Has been persecuted along with other shag species for alleged destruction of large numbers of fresh water fish. Partially protected.

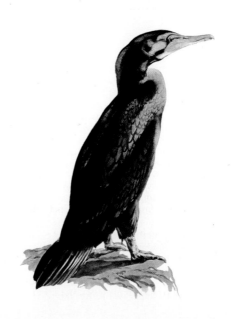

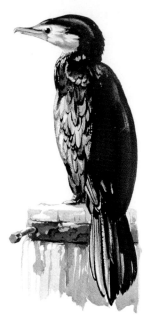

LITTLE SHAG (Kawaupaka)
Phalacrocorax melanoleucos

Size	56cm.
Status:	Fairly common.
Range:	Throughout main islands. Also Australia and Melanesia.
Habitat:	Fresh water, mountain areas, coastal areas.
Description:	Adults are black with spots of white common on the throat and foreneck. Immature birds are completely black or brownish black. Short yellow bills and black feet.
Food:	Similar to black shag.
Voice:	Deep croak.
Breeding:	Seasons vary. Three to four bluish eggs.
General:	Closely related to the Australian little pied shag, it is the most commonly seen shag, and the smallest. Also called the white-throated shag. Fully protected.

WHITE-FACED HERON (Blue Crane)
Ardea novaehollandiae

Size:	66cm.
Status:	Fairly common.
Range:	On main islands, most off-shore islands, including Campbell Island. Also Australia, New Guinea, Indonesia.
Habitat:	Spreads from coastal areas inland, it favours lake margins, rivers and estuaries, also open spaces.
Description:	Dark bluish grey crown, white strip over and behind eyes, long black bill. Body is bluish grey with under parts greyish pink. Legs yellowish.
Food:	Insects, fish and frogs.
Voice:	Gutteral sound.
Breeding:	December-June. Three to five blue-green eggs.
General:	Since migrating to New Zealand in the 1940's this Australian bird has become well-established, preferring open to forest country. Fully protected.

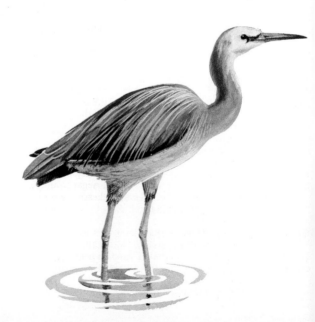

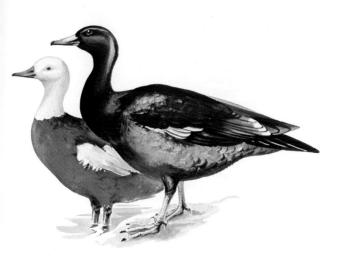

PARADISE DUCK (Putangitangi)

Tadorna variegata

Size:	63cm.
Status:	Common where protected.
Range:	Distributed widely in band from Taranaki to Gisborne, in Northland and the South Island especially on the eastern side of the Southern Alps.
Habitat:	River flats, grassy plains, mountain valleys, occasionally in coastal regions.
Description:	In contrast to most birds, the female is almost as colourful as the male with white head and neck. The male has a black head with bluish green hue. Both sexes have dark backs with variegated body colours elsewhere. The female has a chestnut under body, the male is basically dark.
Food:	Grasses, herbs and insects.
Voice:	The male has a deep discordant warning cry while the female has a high pitched call.
Breeding:	August-January. Six to twelve cream coloured eggs.
General:	As nesting sites it prefers hollow trees and clay banks in back country areas. Regarded as a game bird. Protected in some districts.

GREY DUCK (Parera)

Anas superciliosa

Size:	55cm.
Status:	Common.
Range:	Widely distributed throughout main islands and off-shore islands.
Habitat:	All types of country from coastal to sub-alpine, wherever fresh waters are to be found.
Description:	Two conspicuous cream stripes outline the eyes, the bill is lead colour, the legs and feet yellowish brown. Both sexes are alike in having greyish brown plumage.
Food:	Plant and animal matter - insects, seeds, shellfish, seaweed etc.
Voice:	Characteristic quacking sound.
Breeding:	August-December. Five to ten cream-green eggs.
General:	Our commonest species of duck, the grey duck is often confused with the mallard. Whilst the mallard is a sedentary species, the grey duck travels extensively, movements of one thousand kilometres are not uncommon. A game bird. Protected, except in open season.

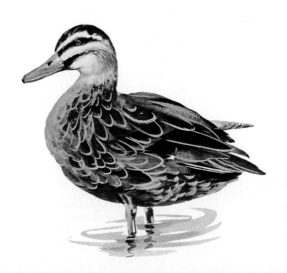

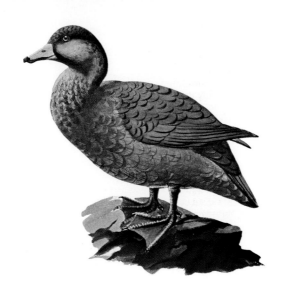

BLUE DUCK (Whio)
Hymenolaimus malacorhychos

Size:	53cm.
Status:	Uncommon.
Range:	North Island south of Coromandel Peninsula, northern and western districts of the South Island.
Habitat:	Rivers and streams of mountainous and hilly regions where there is a native forest cover.
Description:	Dove grey plumage with metallic gloss to head. Narrow white bill, dark brown feet. The chest is spotted walnut and both sexes are alike, other than the male is slightly larger than the female.
Food:	Aquatic insects and larvae.
Voice:	Male a husky whistle "whio", female a croaking, rather drawn out call "craark".
Breeding:	August-November. Four to nine creamy white eggs.
General:	Once much more widely distributed but seriously affected by the destruction and modification of mountain forests. Fully protected.

NEW ZEALAND SCAUP (Papango) (Black Teal)
Aythya novaeseelandiae

Size:	40cm.
Status:	Fairly common.
Range:	Throughout main islands.
Habitat:	Prefers large and open waters, lagoons and lakes.
Description:	The male has a black head with patches of purple and green sheen. Its body is brownish black on the upper parts and dark brown on the under parts and legs. The male has a conspicuous yellow eye, the female a brown eye. Plumage of the female is duller and lacks gloss.
Food:	Small aquatic animals and seeds from the lake floors.
Voice:	Male isssues a soft whistling sound, female more liquid.
Breeding:	October-March. Five to eight creamy white eggs.
General:	Of chubby shape, the scaup is also known as the black teal. It is an expert diver, often going down six to ten feet. Fully protected.

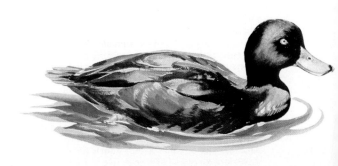

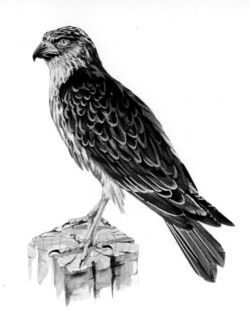

AUSTRALIAN HARRIER (Kahu) (Hawk)

Circus approximans

Size:	60cm.
Status:	Fairly common.
Range:	Throughout main islands, seen also at Auckland and Campbell Islands. Australia and Melanesia.
Habitat:	Fern-clad hills, open plains, swamps, scrub country.
Description:	Dark brown plumage in adults, under parts buff colour. Young birds are darker, their plumage lightening with age. Legs are yellow. Face has owl-like appearance common to all harriers.
Food:	Insects, mice, frogs, lizards, bird eggs, dead stock found on highways and elsewhere.
Voice:	"Kee Kee Kee" sound during courtship displays.
Breeding:	October-December. Three to five white eggs.
General:	Soars in wide circles with wings tipped upwards, differs from New Zealand's other hawk, the falcon, by being slower and more leisurely, rather than fierce and aggressive. Partially protected.

11

NEW ZEALAND FALCON (Kararea) (Bush Haw

Falco novaeseelandiae

Size:	41-48cm.
Status:	Fairly common.
Range:	Throughout main islands but rare north of the volcanic plateau of the central North Island. Some off-shore and outlying islands.
Habitat:	Native forests, more particularly in hilly districts.
Description:	Females are slightly larger than males but both are only half the size of the harrier. Head and upper parts are greyish black with under parts pale tawny to reddish brown. Legs are yellow, claws greyish black. The young are darker.
Food:	Birds and small mammals.
Voice:	A staccato call "Kek-Kek-Kek-Kek" repeated at short intervals. Also a shrill scream when flying.
Breeding:	October-December. Two to four eggs, reddish brown with chocolate blotches.
General:	Also known as the bush hawk the falcon is seen today mainly in the high country having been driven away from the habitat of man for its fierce predatory nature. Fully protected.

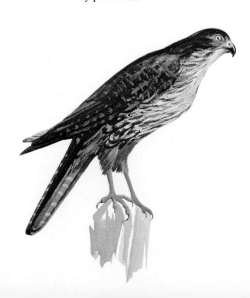

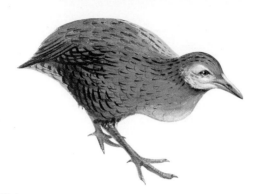

WEKA (Woodhen)
Gallirallus australis

Size:	54cm.
Status:	Fairly common.
Range:	North Island; Poverty Bay and a few scattered localities where re-introduced. South Island: from Nelson and northern Marlborough to Fiordland and West Otago. Stewart Island. Introduced to some off-shore islands and the Chathams.
Habitat:	Native forest and scrub, some urban areas and farmland.
Description:	There are four subspecies of weka; North island, South Island, Stewart Island and Bluff. Differences are mainly in variations in the toning and amount of black and brown in the plumage. In addition, very dark forms of the South Island and Stewart Island subspecies are common.
Food:	Animal and vegetable matter of great variety, including small birds and mammals.
Voice:	A shrill whistle "coo-et" repeated many times. Also a deep drumming note.
Breeding:	September-April. Three to six eggs, creamy white or pinkish with brown and purplish blotches.
General:	A flightless bird of the rail family, the weka is the size of a small hen. Is is as much nocturnal as diurnal, becoming more active at dusk. It has a deserved reputation among trampers as a thief, for it will seize any shiny object. Fully protected, except on Chatham Islands.

PUKEKO (Swamphen)
Porphyrio porphyrio

Size:	51cm.
Status:	Common.
Range:	Throughout main islands and some outlying islands.
Habitat:	Swamp areas, river banks, lagoons and open scrub wetlands.
Description:	Head, neck and upper parts are shiny, sooty black with touches of green. Bright blue under parts, long legs and feet of pale red. Large bright red bill.
Food:	Mainly vegetarian, also grass grubs, snails, insects.
Voice:	A screeching "kwee-ow" acts as an alarm call. There are also mating and contact calls.
Breeding:	August-March. Four to eight blotchy buff eggs.
General:	Whilst the pukeko may walk awkwardly with frequent head jerks, it can run well and at high speed. It flies strongly with rapid wing beats. A game bird. Protected in some districts.

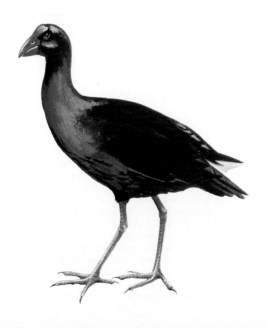

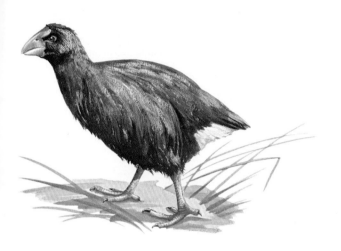

TAKAHE
Notornis mantelli

Size:	63cm.
Status:	Very rare.
Range:	Confined to Fiordland, west of Lake Te Anau.
Habitat:	Glacial valley floors, tussock country.
Description:	Head, neck and under parts iridescent indigo blue. Back and upper tail olive green, under tail white. Scarlet and pink beak, red legs and feet.
Food:	Tussock shoots, leaves, grass seeds and insects.
Voice:	A short "klowp" note and an "oomf" alarm note. Similar to a weka.
Breeding:	October-March. One or two eggs of dull cream colour, with brown and mauve blotches.
General:	A flightless bird, considered extinct until rediscovered in 1948. Has been bred in captivity with success at Mount Bruce, Wairarapa, but must still be considered an endangered species. Fully protected.

AUSTRALIAN COOT
Fulica atra

Size:	38cm.
Status:	Common.
Range:	Volcanic central plateau and southern parts of North Island. Canterbury and Otago in the South Island. Also Australia.
Habitat:	Inland lakes and reed-lined ponds of good size.
Description:	Plumage is black, being darkest at head and neck, brownish black on under parts. Bill is oyster white, legs and feet olive green to grey.
Food:	Underwater weeds, insects.
Voice:	Harsh metallic sound, also "Krat, Krat"grunt.
Breeding:	August-December. Five to seven cream coloured eggs.
General:	First appearing in numbers in the 1950's, the coot has spread rapidly on both main islands, wherever open waters are to be found. Fully protected.

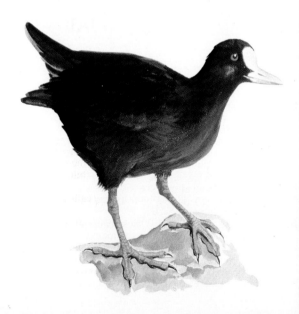

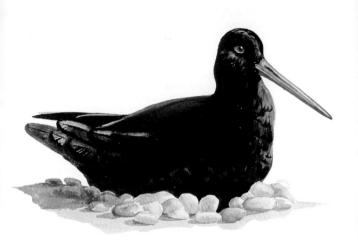

OYSTERCATCHER (VARIABLE)
(Torea) (Northern Oystercatcher)
Haematopus unicolor

Size:	48cm.
Status:	Common.
Range:	Throughout main islands and most off-shore islands.
Habitat:	Sandy beaches, rocky coasts, dry river beds.
Description:	There are two colour phases - the black with glossy brownish-black upper parts and slightly lighter underparts; and the pied, with brownish-black upper parts, white under parts with some white markings on the wing tips. Long crimson bill, red legs.
Food:	Shellfish and crustacea.
Voice:	A long series of piping mating calls and a shrill "Kee-eep" note, among others.
Breeding:	October-January. Three pale brown eggs with blackish blotches.
General:	A similar species is the South Island Oystercatcher which has black and white colourings, much as the pied phase of the variable oystercatcher. Fully protected.

BANDED DOTTEREL (Tuturiwhatu) (Mountain Pl〔

Charadrius bicinctus

Size:	18cm.
Status:	Common.
Range:	Throughout main islands, off-shore islands, also in Tasmania and Australia. Migratory within New Zealand, spending the winter months in the North Island(some also migrating to Australia), then returning for the summer to the South Island.
Habitat:	River beds, coastal beaches, lake shorelines.
Description:	Greyish brown on back, with black bill. Under parts are white with bands of black and chestnut which tend to fade markedly between February and May.
Food:	Mainly insects.
Voice:	Call is close to Maori name "Tuturiwhatu".
Breeding:	August-December. Two to three greenish yellow eggs, heavily spotted dark brown and black.
General:	Travels widely in large flocks from coast to coast and from South to North Island after breeding time. Fully protected.

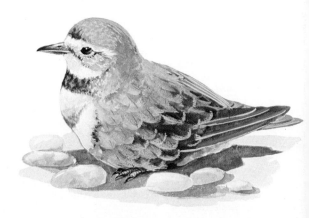

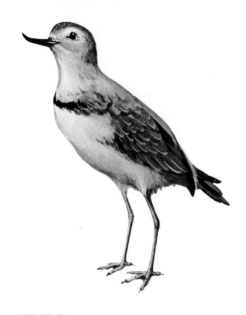

WRYBILL (Ngutu parore) (Wrybilled Plover)
Anarhynchus frontalis

Size:	20cm.
Status:	Fairly common.
Range:	Breeds in Canterbury and Otago in the South Island and winters in the northern parts of the North Island.
Habitat:	Shingle river beds in the South Island, mudflats and lakes in the North Island.
Description:	Medium grey head and back, all white under parts, except during breeding season when a band of black adorns the upper breast. Long black bill with unique curve to right. Blackish grey legs.
Food:	Mainly insects.
Voice:	A piping whistle is characteristic call.
Breeding:	September-November. Two pale blue eggs with fine speckled spots of darker hues.
General:	A tiny bird which runs, swims and flies rapidly. Nests among the larger stones of river shingle. Fully protected.

GODWIT (Kuaka)
Limosa lapponica

Size:	40cm.
Status:	Common.
Range:	Throughout main islands and Chatham Islands. Occasional visitor to other outlying islands. Also, Northern Europe, Asia, Africa and Middle East.
Habitat:	Mudflats and tidal zones.
Description:	Speckled brown upper parts during the breeding season, lighter brown underneath. Outside breeding months, speckled brown grey upper parts and white under parts. Long slender upturned black bill and grey-black legs.
Food:	Small sea animals and shellfish.
Voice:	Continuous twittering whilst in flight and on nests.
Breeding:	May-June in Alaska and Eastern Siberia. Four olive-brown eggs.
General:	Godwits migrate in flocks of thousands in August and remain in New Zealand until March-April. Fully protected.

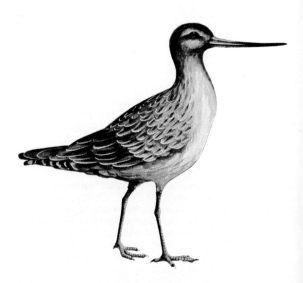

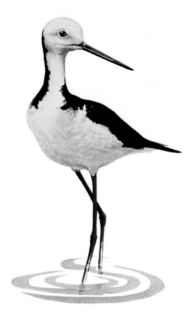

PIED STILT (Poaka) (Barker)
Himantopus himantopus

Size:	38cm.
Status:	Common.
Range:	Throughout main islands. Also Australia, New Guinea, Indonesia and Phillipines.
Habitat:	Inland swamps and lakes, tidal mudflats, marshes.
Description:	Small-bodied wader with long slender light red legs. Back, wings and back of head are black, front of head and all under parts are white. The long slight bill is black in colour.
Food:	Small marine life, molluscs and worms.
Voice:	Yelps continuously like a small puppy.
Breeding:	June-February North Island, September-February South Island. Four buff to olive-brown eggs.
General:	The pied stilt migrates within New Zealand from inland breeding areas to the coast, many from the South Island to the North for the winter period. Fully protected.

NEW ZEALAND PIGEON (Kereru)
Hemiphaga novaeseelandiae

Size:	51cm.
Status:	Common.
Range:	Throughout main islands and off-shore islands.
Habitat:	Native forest, including much modified remnants and adjacent exotic vegetation, rare in beech forest.
Description:	Head and upper parts are coppery iridescent green and violet. Tail above is greenish black and below light grey. Under parts from the upper breast down are white. The bill, legs and feet are shades of red.
Food:	Fruit and foliage.
Voice:	A soft "Kuu" uttered singly and with fairly long pauses between.
Breeding:	November-January. One white egg.
General:	This large plump pigeon has a tame nature and can readily be approached. It moves noisily from bush to bush in the forest, feeding on the fruit of many native and exotic species. A subspecies is present but very rare on the Chatham Islands. Fully protected.

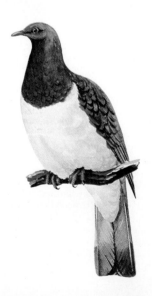

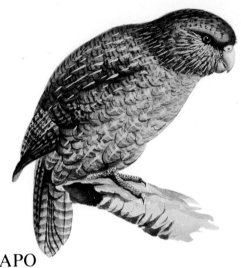

KAKAPO
Strigops habroptilus

Size:	56-66cm.
Status:	Very rare.
Range:	A few valleys in the Milford Sound region, Fiordland and Stewart Island.
Habitat:	Native forest, sub-alpine and alpine zones.
Description:	A heavy-bodied parrot with moss-green plumage streaked with brown on the upper parts. Brownish tinges on the under parts. Bill yellowish, feet greyish. Flightless, but a good climber.
Food:	Leaves, stems, roots and fruits of a wide range of vegetation.
Voice:	A series of low but resonant booms repeated at intervals, probably restricted to the breeding season. Also a variety of grunts and screams.
Breeding:	December-February. Two to four white eggs.
General:	Once plentiful in both islands the kakapo must now be considered in grave danger of extinction. Recent evidence suggests a continued decline in numbers and range. A small colony exists on Stewart Island with breeding taking place and a few birds are held on Maud Island, Marlborough Sounds in an attempt to preserve the species. Fully protected.

KAKA
Nestor meridionalis

Size:	43-48cm.
Status:	Fairly common.
Range:	Throughout main islands and the larger off-shore islands.
Habitat:	Large areas of native forest and occasionally adjacent exotic vegetation and nearby isolated patches of bush, particularly podocarps.
Description:	The North Island subspecies of this large parrot has olive brown plumage with a reddish tinge to the under parts. Heavy slate grey bill and dark grey feet. The South Island subspecies is brighter hued.
Food:	Fruit, leaves, insects and nectar.
Voice:	A harsh "Kaka" also many whistling, musical notes.
Breeding:	November-January. Four to five white eggs.
General:	There is a North Island and a South Island subspecies, the South Island birds being rather more brightly coloured. The kaka avoids settled districts, it is confined to native forest areas. It flies directly at considerable height and speed; on the ground it has a hopping motion. Fully protected.

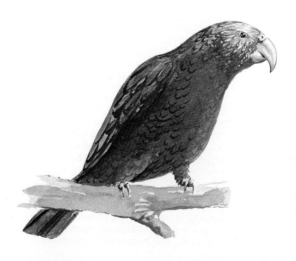

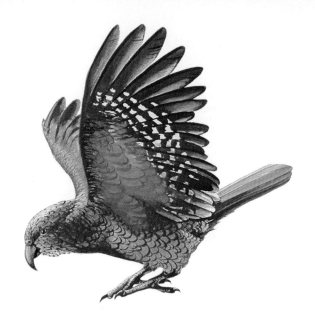

KEA
Nestor notabilis

Size:	46-48cm.
Status:	Common.
Range:	South Island high country from Marlborough and Nelson to Fiordland. Straying to coastal areas.
Habitat:	Native forest and the sub-alpine and alpine zones.
Description:	Body is dull green with blue-green tail feathers; crimson patches under the wings. Bill is longer than the kaka's and is dark grey as are the feet.
Food:	Leaves, buds, fruit, insects and carrion.
Voice:	A penetrating and drawn out "Keaa" and a variety of softer calls.
Breeding:	July-January. Two to four white eggs.
General:	This parrot has been persecuted as a sheep killer but there is some doubt as to the extent it attacks healthy animals. Partially protected (may be hunted or killed by an occupier of land only when causing damage on that land). Fully protected.

RED-CROWNED PARAKEET (Kakariki)
Cyanoramphus novaezelandiae

Size:	Male 27-30cm, female 23-27cm.
Status:	Rare on mainland, common on off-shore islands.
Range:	A few localities throughout the main islands; many off-shore islands. Subspecies on the Kermadec, Chatham, Antipodes and Norfolk Islands.
Habitat:	Native forest (on mainland, only the more extensive forests).
Description:	Notable for red patches on forehead, behind eyes and on rump. Body is grass green on upper parts and yellowish green on under parts. Feet greyish brown.
Food:	Fruits, seeds, leaves and buds.
Voice:	A rapid "Ki-Ki-Ki-Ki" in flight, also a variety of chattering and soft, musical calls.
Breeding:	October-March. Four to nine white eggs.
General:	Three other parakeets occur: the yellow-crowned parakeet (also illustrated), the orange-fronted parakeet (now very rare) and the Antipodes Island parakeet (largest of the species). Fully protected.

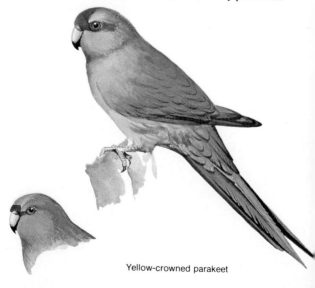

Yellow-crowned parakeet

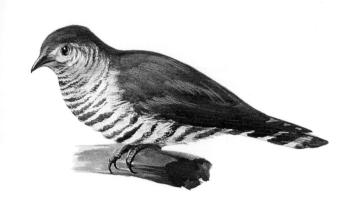

SHINING CUCKOO (Pipiwharauroa) (Whistler)
Chrysococcyx lucidus

Size:	16cm.
Status:	Common.
Range:	Throughout the main islands and many off-shore islands from September to March. Winters in the Solomon Islands and Bismark Archipelago.
Habitat:	Native and exotic forest and almost everywhere else provided there is some tree or shrub cover and a host species (preferably grey warbler) is present.
Description:	Slightly larger than the house sparrow. Body is a bright green on the upper parts, changing to golden tint. Under parts are white with coppery-green bands.
Food:	Mainly insects.
Voice:	An often repeated "Kiu-Kiu-Kiu" with the last two notes ending with a downward, slurred intonation. Also a single note "Tsui" repeated several times.
Breeding:	Lays eggs in nest of grey warbler and sometimes fantail, tomtit, silvereye and others. Eggs greenish or bluish white to olive brown or dark greenish brown.
General:	Rarely seen but their ventriloquistic notes are distinctive. Fully protected.

LONG-TAILED CUCKOO (Koekoea)
Eudynemys taitsensis

Size:	40cm.
Status:	Common.
Range:	Throughout main islands and many off-shore islands October to March. Winters in the North Pacific.
Habitat:	Native and exotic forests.
Description:	Much larger than the shining cuckoo. Head and upper parts of the body are speckled dark brown, under parts are buff with dark streaks.
Food:	Insects, small lizards.
Voice:	A long drawn out screech "zzwheet" with a rising emphasis. Alarm call a succession of rapid twittering notes "zzip-zip-zip". Often heard calling at night.
Breeding:	Lays eggs in nests of several species but principally the whitehead in the North Island and the yellowhead and brown creeper in the South Island and Stewart Island. Eggs creamy white with spots or blotches in shades of browns and greys.
General:	Like the shining cuckoo, this bird is heard more than seen. Both cuckoos are parasitic, laying their eggs in the nests of both native and exotic species. Fully protected.

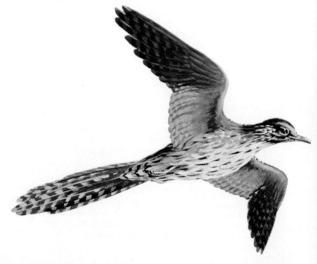

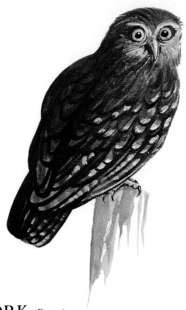

MOREPORK (Ruru)
Ninox novaeseelandiae

Size:	29cm.
Status:	Common.
Range:	Throughout main islands and many off-shore and outlying islands.
Habitat:	Native and exotic forests, also small patches of modified forest and exotic trees.
Description:	Head and back are dark brown, wings are tipped with white. Triangular spots of brown appear on light brown under parts. Bill is white on the ridge, feet are dark brown.
Food:	Insects, small mammals, birds and lizards.
Voice:	"Morepork" sometimes repeated and prolonged, and a variety of screechs and mewing calls.
Breeding:	October-November. Two to three white eggs.
General:	The native owl with the distinctive call is sometimes seen at dusk in suburban gardens. Fully protected.

KINGFISHER (Kotare)

Halcyon sancta

Size:	24cm.
Status:	Common.
Range:	Throughout the main islands, especially in the north. Also most off-shore islands.
Habitat:	Haunts open country, near the sea, fresh water streams and forest clearings.
Description:	Bill is black, dark blue-green colour above the eye, buff-white below the eye and on under parts. Back is sea green, wings and tail blue-green. Legs are dark brown.
Food:	Grubs, mice, lizards, fish, crabs, small insects.
Voice:	Usually silent. Call and alarm note are piercing "Kik Kik".
Breeding:	October-January. Four or five white eggs.
General:	The kingfisher makes its nest by boring into a rotten tree or excavating a tunnel in a clay bank. The eggs are laid on the wood or earth without nesting materials. Fully protected.

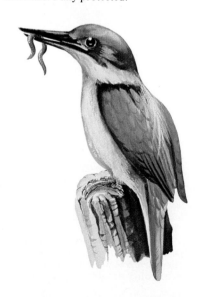

Male

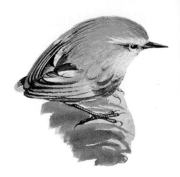

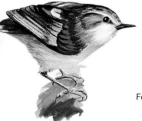
Female

RIFLEMAN (Titipounamu)
Acanthisitta chloris

Size:	8cm.
Status:	Fairly common.
Range:	Southern two thirds of the North Island and throughout the South Island and Stewart Island. A few off-shore islands.
Habitat:	Native and exotic forests and scrub-land.
Description:	The male has a dark brown bill, green back, yellow rump, and white under parts. The female differs in that its back is brown with buff on under parts.
Food:	Insects, obtained from the bark, mosses and lichens of the larger trees.
Voice:	A high-pitched "zipt", singly or rapidly repeated.
Breeding:	August-January. Two to four white eggs.
General:	The smallest bird in New Zealand. North Island and South Island birds are regarded as separate subspecies but the differences are slight. Fully protected.

WELCOME SWALLOW
Hirundo tahitica

Size:	15cm.
Status:	Common.
Range:	Throughout main islands, more common in North Island up to mountain areas. Also some outlying islands.
Habitat:	Open country, farm and urban areas.
Description:	Reddish-chestnut tinge to forehead and throat, back is dark blue, wings and forked tail dark brown.
Food:	Insects, especially over water.
Voice:	A twittering call.
Breeding:	August-February. Three to five white eggs, speckled brown.
General:	Migrated from Australia and the South Pacific from the 1950's, the bird has become well established in a short space of time. Fully protected.

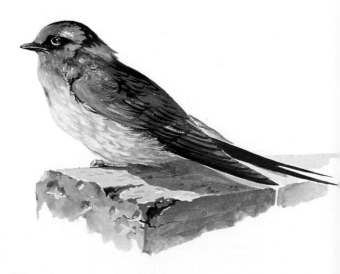

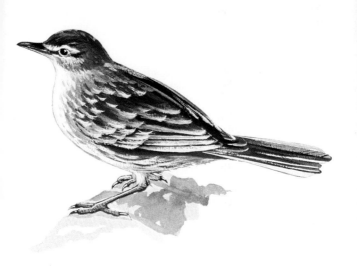

NEW ZEALAND PIPIT (Pihoihoi)
Anthus novaeseelandiae

Size:	19cm.
Status:	Common.
Range:	Throughout main islands and most off-shore and outlying islands. Subspecies on Antipodes, Auckland and Chatham Islands.
Habitat:	Scrub country in the lowlands, river beds, tussock country in the sub-alpine areas.
Description:	Light brown and speckled like a skylark, which it resembles. Under parts are white with two white outer feathers on each side of the brown tail.
Food:	Insects, caterpillers, sometimes seeds.
Voice:	A short trilling "peet peet" call.
Breeding:	August-March. Three to four cream eggs, blotched and spotted brown.
General:	First discovered in Queen Charlotte Sound by Captain Cook's second voyage. Fully protected.

WHITEHEAD (Popokatea)
Mohoua albicilla

Size:	15cm.
Status:	Fairly common.
Range:	Southern two thirds of the North Island, Great Barrier, Little Barrier, and Kapiti Islands.
Habitat:	Native forest and exotic pine forest up to 1200m.
Description:	Head and under parts are white with brown tinge. Back, rump and tail are brown. Bill and feet black.
Food:	Insects and fruits.
Voice:	The song has a similarity to the opening notes of a chaffinch song. Also single "zit" note or several in succession.
Breeding:	October-February. Two to four eggs, white or pinkish with brown, reddish brown or red spots.
General:	Usually moves about the forest in small groups. The yellowhead (also illustrated) is of the same family and is now confined to South Island native beech forests. Both fully protected.

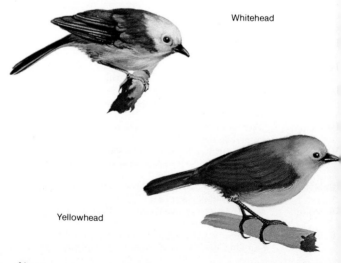

Whitehead

Yellowhead

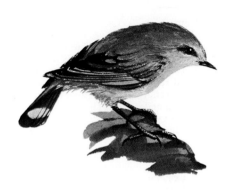

GREY WARBLER (Riroriro)
Gerygone igata

Size:	11cm.
Status:	Common.
Range:	Throughout main islands and many off-shore islands.
Habitat:	Native and exotic forests and almost everywhere else provided there is some tree or shrub cover.
Description:	A small greyish brown bird with a short rounded tail. An identifying feature are the white tail tips seen when the bird is in flight.
Food:	Insects and spiders usually obtained from tree bark, leaves and twigs.
Voice:	A sweet, high pitched, warbling call of varying length. Sometimes a short call of three notes preceding the main song.
Breeding:	August-December. Three to five eggs, pinkish white with reddish brown spots.
General:	More often heard than seen. The most preferred host of the shining cuckoo. A similar warbler on the Chatham Islands is regarded as a separate species. Fully protected.

FANTAIL (Piwakawaka)
Rhipidura fuliginosa

Size:	16cm.
Status:	Common.
Range:	Throughout the main islands and off-shore islands. Also Australia and the Pacific.
Habitat:	Forests of all types and many man-made enviroments providing trees and shrubs.
Description:	The North Island species is dark brown above and buff on under parts. The South Island fantail is black above and choclate brown underneath. The long spread tail makes identification simple.
Food:	Insects caught in the air during short erratic flights.
Voice:	Usual call a high pitched, repeated "cheet". A succession of these with variations produce its song.
Breeding:	August-January. Three to four eggs, cream with grey and brown spots.
General:	North Island, South Island and Chatham Island subspecies. A black form is common in the South Island subspecies. Fully protected.

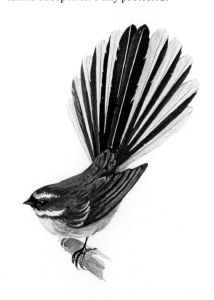

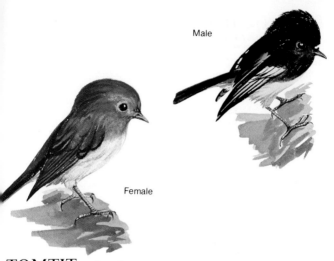

Male

Female

TOMTIT (Miromiro)
Petroica macrocephala

Size:	13cm.
Status:	Fairly common.
Range:	Throughout main islands and some off-shore and outlying islands.
Habitat:	Native and exotic forests.
Description:	There are five subspecies; North Island, South Island, Chatham Island, Auckland Island and Snares Island. North Island male has pure white underparts and the female greyish white underparts. The South and Chatham Islands birds have yellowish breast and abdomen.
Food:	Insects obtained from tree trunks and branches and the forest floor.
Voice:	Male a high pitched "swee", female a faint "seet", Song a high pitched trill "weedli-weedli-weedli".
Breeding:	August-February. (Usually two broods reared). Three to four eggs, cream with yellowish and purplish brown spots.
General:	This bird usually keeps to a defined territory in the forest and gives a distinctive and aggressive performance when intruders appear. Fully protected.

ROBIN (Toutouwai)
Petroica australis

Size:	18cm.
Status:	Fairly common.
Range:	Central and southern North Island, South Island, Stewart Island and some off-shore islands.
Habitat:	Native and exotic forests and scrub land.
Description:	North Island and Stewart Island birds have ivory white underparts, South Island birds are slightly larger and have a yellowish breast.
Food:	Insects.
Voice:	A strong "Twit-twit-twit" repeated many times, and a wide variety of other musical and chirping notes.
Breeding:	August-February. Two to four eggs, cream with purplish brown spots.
General:	Like the tomtit, the robin is belligerent in defending its territory and it will zigzag around an intruder emitting staccato alarm notes to discourage him. Fully protected.

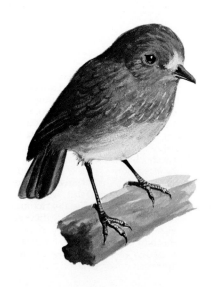

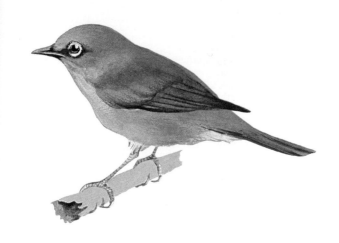

SILVEREYE (Tahou) (Waxeye)
Zosterops lateralis

Size:	12cm.
Status:	Common.
Range:	Throughout main islands and many off-shore and outlying islands. Also Australia.
Habitat:	Native and exotic forest to some extent but mainly open country with some tree cover.
Description:	Upper parts bright yellowish-olive green colour with eye ringed in white. Wing and tail feathers brown, under parts greyish chestnut shades.
Food:	Insects, fruit and nectar.
Voice:	A warbling, continuous song made up of trills, slurs, and other high pitched notes. A common flocking call is "cree".
Breeding:	August-February. Two, sometimes three broods in a season. Three to four pale blue eggs.
General:	Has become common only in the last hundred years. Partially protected. (may be hunted or killed by an occupier of land only when causing damage on that land).

BELLBIRD (Korimako)
Anthornis melanura

Size:	20cm.
Status:	Common.
Range:	Throughout main islands and many off-shore islands.
Habitat:	Native forest and scrubland, also exotic forests and exotic vegetation near native forest.
Description:	This bird has olive green colouring, the male with a purple gloss on the head and a tuft of yellowish wing feathers. Under parts are yellow-green. The female has duller plumage, a white stripe below the eye and yellow-brown under parts. The iris of the male is red, that of the female brown.
Food:	Nectar, fruit and insects.
Voice:	A wide variety of liquid notes, clicks and other sounds of a bell-like quality. Sometimes an often repeated bell note. Alarm call a repeated, harsh "Pek-pek-pek".
Breeding:	September-January. Three to four eggs, pinkish brown spots and blotches.
General:	A slightly different form occurs on the Three Kings Islands. Fully protected.

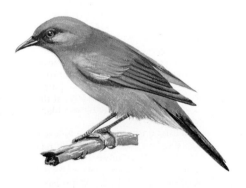

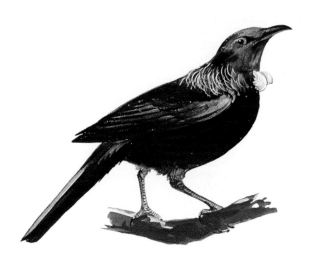

TUI (Parson Bird)
Prosthemadera novaeseelandiae

Size:	Male 32cm, female 29cm.
Status:	Common.
Range:	Throughout main islands and many off-shore and outlying islands.
Habitat:	Native forest, particularly podocarp and broadleaf; and exotic vegetation adjacent to native forest.
Description:	Metallic dark green and blue plumage for both sexes. Distinctive pair of white tufts at throat, white spots on wings. Bill and feet brown-black.
Food:	Nectar, insects and fruit.
Voice:	Song resembles bellbird's but is stronger and more resonant. Alarm call is a harsh, repeated "Keer-keer".
Breeding:	November-January. Three to four eggs, white or pale pink with reddish brown specks or blotches.
General:	A subspecies on the Chatham Islands is slightly larger. Fully protected.

KOKAKO (Wattled Crow)
Callaeas cinerea

Size:	37cm.
Status:	Fairly rare.
Range:	North Auckland and central North Island; possibly a few scattered localities in the South Island.
Habitat:	Native forest with a more or less continuous canopy, particularly where there are emergent podocarps.
Description:	Dark bluish grey bird with long black legs and bright blue wattles at the throat. Under parts ash grey, tinged with brown.
Food:	Leaves, flowers and fruits.
Voice:	A variety of rich organ like notes and bell like calls, usually of descending pitch. The alarm call is rather similar to the tui's.
Breeding:	November-March. Two to three eggs, pale brownish-grey with brown and purplish brown.
General:	Once widely distributed, the kokako has declined considerably in the last hundred years. The South Island subspecies, which has orange wattles, has rarely been seen in recent years. Fully protected.

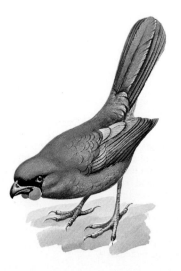

North Island

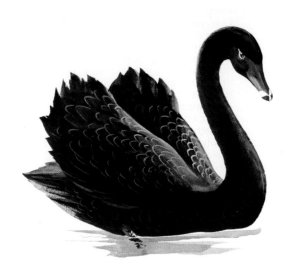

BLACK SWAN
Cygnus atratus

Size:	100cm.
Status:	Fairly common.
Range:	Throughout main islands and Chatham Islands. Introduced from Australia.
Habitat:	Lakes, coastal estuaries and bays.
Description:	Large black bird with a rose-red bill which has a broad white band crossing it. White on the wings, legs black. Has longer neck and is darker than the Canada Goose.
Food:	Water vegetation of all kinds.
Voice:	Has plaintive sustained musical note.
Breeding:	June-December. Four to seven greenish white eggs.
General:	Partially protected, (may be hunted in the season in some districts).

CANADA GOOSE
Branta canadensis

Size:	100cm.
Status:	Common.
Range:	Well established in Canterbury and Otago, rare in North Island.
Habitat:	High country valleys, lagoons, South Island lakes.
Description:	Similar in size to the black swan. Has a glossy black head and neck with white band from throat to eye. Body is brown on upper parts and light brown on under parts. Tail and rump are black.
Food:	Graze on grasses.
Voice:	Shrill "honk honk".
Breeding:	October-December. Four to seven creamy white eggs.
General:	A game bird. Not protected.

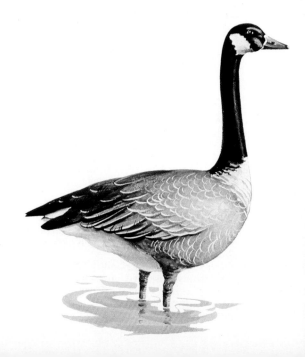

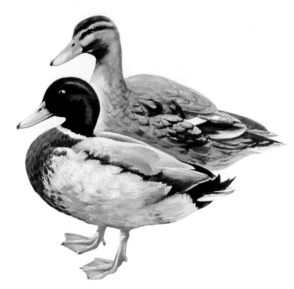

MALLARD
Anas platyrynchos

Size:	58cm.
Status:	Common.
Range:	Throughout main islands an Chatham Islands. Introduced from the British Isles.
Habitat:	All types of county from coastal to sub-alpine; wherever fresh waters are found.
Description:	The male has a dark green head, white collar, brownish grey back, purple breast and grey under parts. Curled tail feathers are black, rest are white. The female is very similar in appearance to the grey duck, but is browner and lacks the characteristic facial stripes.
Food:	Both plant and animal - insects, seeds, shellfish, etc.
Voice:	Female has duck "quack", male is higher pitched.
Breeding:	August-December. Eight to twenty greenish white eggs.
General:	Protected, (except in open season).

CALIFORNIA QUAIL
Lophortyx californica

Size:	25cm.
Status:	Common.
Range:	Throughout the main islands and Chatham Islands, Also North America and elsewhere.
Habitat:	Edge and cut-over areas of exotic forests, scrub country and farmland where there is suitable tree and scrub cover.
Description:	Grey head with black crest facing forward in the male, white band traversing from eye to round chin, black throat. Back green-brown, tail grey. Upper breast slate grey, sides brown with white patches. The female has shorter crest and is browner all over, no white band from eye to chin.
Food:	Small seeds, soft grasses and occasionally insects.
Voice:	A repeated "Cu-ca-cow" with emphasis on the middle note and a single call "cow" Alarm call is a sharp, staccato "plit, plit, plit".
Breeding:	October-December. Nine to sixteen eggs, cream or buff with brown blotches.
General:	An introduced game bird. Protected, (except in open season).

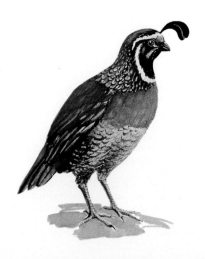

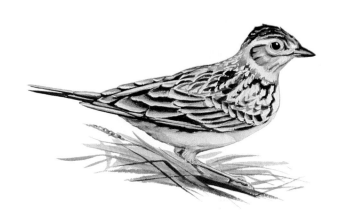

SKYLARK
Alauda arvenis

Size:	18cm.
Status:	Common.
Range:	Throughout main islands and some outlying islands.
Habitat:	Open country up to tussock land.
Description:	Brown to dark brown, upper parts with outer tail feathers white. Head has small crest that can be raised. Buffish white under parts, short bill and light brown legs.
Food:	Insects, seeds.
Voice:	Has a variety of soft notes, both short and sustained.
Breeding:	October-January. Three to seven dirty white eggs.
General:	Often confused with the New Zealand pipit. Not protected.

HEDGE SPARROW
Prunella modularis

Size:	15cm.
Status:	Common.
Range:	Throughout main islands and many off-shore and outlying islands. Also Europe, Scandinavia, Middle East.
Habitat:	All types of country up to the limit of sub-alpine scrub.
Description:	Head is bluish grey, rest of upper parts streaky brown. Under parts vary from white to bluish grey.
Food:	Small seeds and insects obtained on the ground.
Voice:	Call note a penetrating "tseep". Song a rapid, undulating, squeaky warble.
Breeding:	August-January; three to five blue eggs.
General:	An introduced species. Not protected.

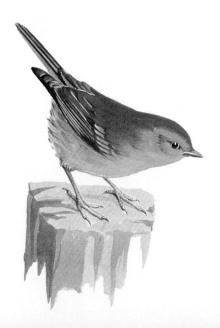

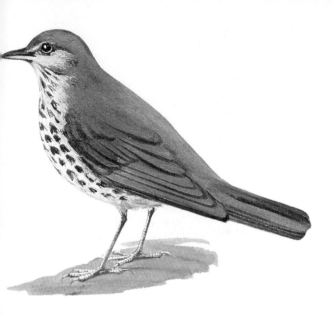

SONG THRUSH
Turdus philomelos

Size:	23cm.
Status:	Common.
Range:	Throughout main islands and most off-shore and outlying islands including sub-antarctic. Also Europe.
Habitat:	All types of country including native and exotic forest.
Description:	Head and upper parts are olive brown. Under parts are whitish with bold dark brown spots. Brown bill and legs.
Food:	Small animal life obtained on the ground, also some fruit and berries.
Voice:	A series of loud, musical, clear-cut notes, often repeated several times.
Breeding:	June-January. Three to five eggs, blue with black spots.
General:	An introduced species. Not protected.

BLACKBIRD
Turdus merula

Size:	25cm.
Status:	Common.
Range:	Throughout main islands and many off-shore and outlying islands including sub-antarctic. Also Europe.
Habitat:	All types of country including dense forest.
Description:	The male is black with an orange bill. The female has dark brown upper parts, a brown bill and lighter brown under parts.
Food:	Earthworms, snails and other small animal life caught on the ground, also a variety of fruit.
Voice:	Similar to the song thrush but notes repetitive and of a more rambling nature. Alarm call a rapid, repeated "Chip-chip-chip".
Breeding:	July-January. Two to four eggs, bluish green with brown speckles.
General:	An introduced species. Not protected.

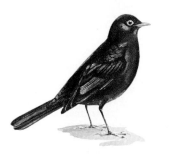

Male

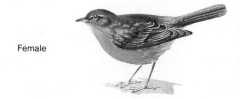

Female

YELLOWHAMMER
Emberiza citrinella *See p. 52*

Size:	16cm.
Status:	Common.
Range:	Throughout main islands and many off-shore and outlying islands.
Habitat:	Pasture lands, marshes, pine plantations and up to tussock country.
Description:	Yellow head, throat and under parts. Back and tail predominately chestnut. The female is less bright in colour.
Food:	Insects, grain.
Voice:	Song rhymes with "little bit of bread and cheese".
Breeding:	October-January. Three to six whitish eggs.
General:	Introduced from Europe in the 1860's. Not protected.

CHAFFINCH
Fringilla coelebs *See p. 52*

Size:	15cm.
Status:	Common.
Range:	Throughout the main islands and many off-shore and outlying islands. Also Europe.
Habitat:	All types of country where there are trees and shrubs. Deep into native and exotic forests.
Description:	Common to male and female are the two white bars on wings and white on tail, otherwise the female is drabber. Crown and nape are greyish blue in the male, mantle and under parts are chestnut, rump greenish. The female has yellowish brown on the crown and nape, with mantle and under parts greyish green.
Food:	Seeds and insects. Also fruits and leaf buds.
Voice:	Song a succession of rattling notes ending with a flourish. Call notes a metallic "pink".
Breeding:	October-February. Four to six eggs, greenish blue with spots and streaks of dark purplish brown.
General:	An introduced species. Not protected.

Yellowhammer

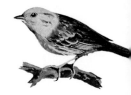

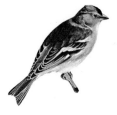

Chaffinch
Male

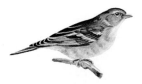

Chaffinch
Female

Greenfinch

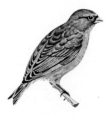

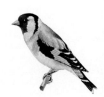

Goldfinch

Myna

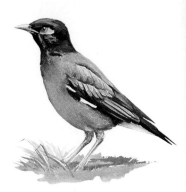

Starling

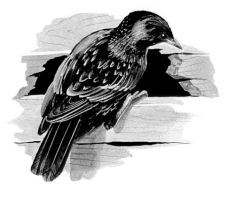

Redpoll

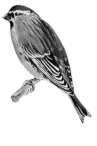

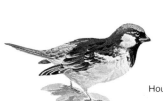

House Sparrow

GREENFINCH
Carduelis chloris *See p. 52*

Size:	15cm.
Status:	Common.
Range:	Throughout the main islands and some off-shore islands. Also Europe, North Africa, Western Asia.
Habitat:	Exotic forests, farmland and urban areas.
Description:	Olive green head, shading to yellowish green on upper parts. Yellowish green under parts, yellow on tail. The female is duller coloured.
Food:	Small seeds and insects. Also fruit, flowers and leaf buds.
Voice:	Call "Chip-chip-duzee". Song "zirr-chea-chee-chee" and variations.
Breeding:	September-January. Four to six eggs, off-white with reddish spots or streaks.
General:	An introduced species. Not protected.

GOLDFINCH
Carduelis carduelis *See p. 52*

Size:	13cm.
Status:	Common.
Range:	Throughout main islands and some off-shore and outlying islands. Also Europe, Asia, Middle East and North Africa.
Habitat:	Exotic forests, farm and urban areas.
Description:	Both sexes have red forehead and throat, white cheeks and brown back. Tail is black with white tips, under parts are white with brown shadings.
Food:	Small seeds and insects. Also leaves and flower buds.
Voice:	High pitched call "pee-yu". Song resembling that of canary but quieter.
Breeding:	September-December. Four to six eggs, bluish white with spots and streaks of reddish brown.
General:	An introduced species. Not protected.

REDPOLL
Carduelis flammea *See p. 53*

Size:	12cm.
Status:	Fairly common.
Range:	Throughout main islands and many off-shore and outlying islands, common on sub-antarctic islands. Also Europe, Asia, North America and Scandinavia.
Habitat:	Very varied, open coastal county to native and exotic forests to above the bush line.
Description:	Red crown, black chin spot, reddish brown wings with long black streaks. Breast and under parts rose to white.
Food:	Small seeds and insects.
Voice:	A metallic twitter "Chuh-chi-chi-chi" in flight also a rippling song.
Breeding:	September-January. Four to six eggs, bluish green spotted and streaked with light brown.
General:	An introduced species. Not protected.

HOUSE SPARROW
Passer domesticus *See p. 53*

Size:	15cm.
Status:	Common.
Range:	Throughout main islands, off-shore and outlying islands, including sub-antarctic.
Habitat:	All types of country, but prefers built-up areas.
Description:	Crown of male is ash grey, chestnut upper parts, black at throat and upper breast, whitish cheeks and under parts. The female is duller brown.
Food:	Seeds and insects. Also grain and fruit.
Voice:	Repeated chirping non-melodic call.
Breeding:	July-April. Five to seven variably spotted white eggs.
General:	An introduced species. Not protected.

STARLING
Sturnus vulgaris
See p. 53

Size: 21cm.
Status: Common.
Range: Throughout main islands, off-shore and outlying islands, including sub-antarctic.
Habitat: Prefers flat settled areas to bush or mountains.
Description: Black plumage with purple and green metallic gloss. In winter time the plumage is speckled with white. Male has yellow bill at breeding time, otherwise black.
Food: Insects, fruit, worms, seaweed.
Voice: Has many tuneful calls and is a good mimic of other birds.
Breeding: August-January. Four to six pale blue eggs.
General: An introduced species. Not protected.

MYNA
Acridotheres tristis
See p. 53

Size: 24cm.
Status: Common.
Range: Found above Wanganui, Palmerston North and Southern Hawkes Bay in the North Island.
Habitat: Near settlements and especially along roadsides.
Description: Greenish black head and neck with bare space around eye. Short, pointed yellow bill, brown upper parts shading to light brown on under parts. White band on wings and tip of tail.
Food: Insects, seeds, fruit.
Voice: Fast sequence of notes from harsh to bell-like.
Breeding: November-February. Three to six pale blue eggs.
General: An introduced species. Not protected.

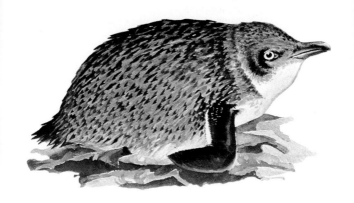

BLUE PENGUIN (Korora)

Eudyptula minor

Size:	40cm.
Status:	Common.
Range:	Throughout main islands, many off-shore and outlying islands. Also Australia.
Habitat:	Sheltered coastal waters.
Description:	There are several sub-species with variable shades of blue on dorsal areas. Sides of face below eye are greyish and under parts are white. Black bill is shorter in male than in female, flippers are black, edged in white.
Food:	Small fish and aquatic life.
Voice:	Sounds range from low purrings to loud screams when disturbed.
Breeding:	August-November. Two white eggs.
General:	Clumsy and nocturnal on land, breeds in hollows, under logs and occasionally under seaside baches. Fully protected.

ROYAL ALBATROSS (Toroa)
Diomedea epomophora

Size:	75-125cm.
Status:	Fairly common.
Range:	Nests on Otago Peninsula, Chatham Islands, Campbell and Auckland Islands, otherwise lives at sea.
Habitat:	Flies over the sea by day, sleeps on water. Nests on mainland at Taiaroa Head, Otago Peninsula.
Description:	White overall except for variable black on upper wings. Bill yellowish, feet yellowish-white.
Food:	Fish.
Voice:	At mating time a series of high, screaming notes; at sea a gutteral croak.
Breeding:	October-January (chick leaves nest in September). One white egg.
General:	Visitors may see this bird at the Taiaroa Head colony controlled by the Otago Peninsula Wildlife Trust. Fully protected.

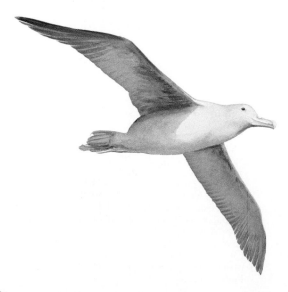

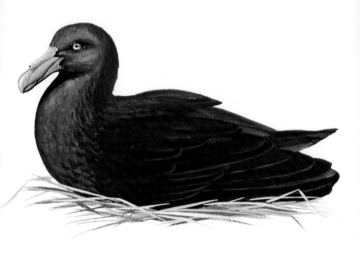

GIANT PETREL
Macronectes giganteus

Size:	65cm.
Status:	Common.
Range:	Throughout main islands and outlying islands, including sub-antarctic islands.
Habitat:	Ocean, estuaries, deep sounds.
Description:	The largest of the petrels. It has a pale brown head with whitish face, bill light brown or greenish. Upper parts of body are dark chocolate brown, fading to light brown on under parts and legs.
Food:	Feeds on fish and carrion.
Voice:	A harsh croak.
Breeding:	August-October. One white egg, freckled brown.
General:	Common to circumpolar Southern Hemisphere. Fully protected.

SOOTY SHEARWATER (Titi) (Muttonbird)
Puffinus griseus

Size:	43cm.
Status:	Common.
Range:	Many off-shore islands, Otago, Westland, Stewart Island and sub-antarctic islands. Also Atlantic and Pacific oceans.
Habitat:	The ocean.
Description:	Sooty brown on upper parts, greyish brown on under parts, tail black.
Food:	Fish and crustacea
Voice:	High pitched rhythmic cry and growling noise that varies from slow to fast tempo.
Breeding:	November-February. One white egg.
General:	Also known as the muttonbird. Protected, except in open season.

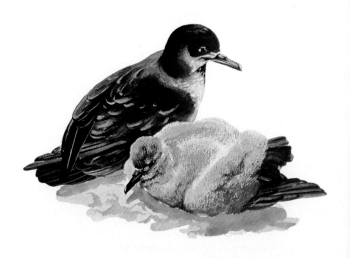

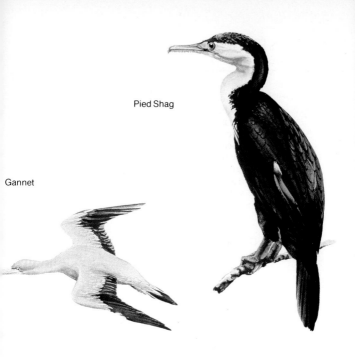

Pied Shag

Gannet

GANNET (Takapu)
Sula serrator

Size: 91cm.
Status: Common.
Range: Large mainland colony at Cape Kidnappers, Hawke Bay, otherwise small off-shore islands of North Island.
Habitat: Coastal waters, bays and harbours.
Description: Upper parts mainly white with yellow head and bluish bill. Tail feathers black, legs dark brown.
Food: Dives for small fish and squid.
Voice: At sea usually silent, at mating time half whistling-half croaking sound.
Breeding: August-December. One chalky white egg.
General: Fully protected.

PIED SHAG (Karuhiruhi)
Phalacrocax varius   *See p. 61*

Size:	81cm.
Status:	Common.
Range:	Throughout main islands and off-shore islands: most occur around the northern coasts of the North Island, the Marlborough Sounds and Stewart Island. Also Australia, Indonesia and Borneo.
Habitat:	Coastal waters, estuaries and lagoons.
Description:	Upper parts including crown are greenish black. Blue circle around eye and bright yellow pouch in front of eye. Sides of face, neck and under parts are white. Black legs.
Food:	Feeds on small fish.
Voice:	Squeals, screams and croaks (like a frog).
Breeding:	August-September/March-April. Two to four pale blue eggs.
General:	Fully protected.

REEF HERON (Matuku moana)
Egretta sacra   *See Back Cover*

Size:	66cm.
Status:	Fairly common.
Range:	Throughout main islands and most off-shore islands. Also Japan and Eastern Pacific.
Habitat:	Rocks under sea cliffs, prefers rocky to sandy coastline.
Description:	Dark slate grey on upper parts, lighter on under parts. Long bill, greyish legs. White strip on throat.
Food:	Feeds on small fish.
Voice:	Gutteral croak.
Breeding:	September-February. Two to three greenish blue eggs.
General:	Fully protected.

RED-BILLED GULL (Tarapunga)
Larus scopulinas   *See Inside Cover*

Size:	37cm.
Status:	Common.
Range:	Throughout main islands and most off-shore islands. Not inland except on Lakes Rotorua and Taupo. Also Australia, New Caledonia and South Africa.
Habitat:	Coasts and occasionally inland.
Description:	Identified by short red bill, red-ringed eye and red feet. Crown of head, nape of neck, under parts and tail are white. First and second tail quills black with white spots. Back is ash grey colour.
Food:	Small fish, shellfish, insects, carrion.
Voice:	High pitched scream plus staccato "Kar kar" cry.
Breeding:	November-January. Two eggs, grey to brown in colour, with variable blotches.
General:	A scavanger of the sea coasts. Fully protected.

BLACK-BILLED GULL (Tarapunga)
Larus bulleri   *See Inside Cover*

Size:	37cm.
Status:	Common.
Range:	South Island rivers and lakes, coasts and cultivated land.
Habitat:	South Island rivers and lakes, coasts and cultivated land.
Description:	Black bill and reddish-black feet. Head, neck, under parts and tail are white. First three tail quills black and white. Pearl grey back.
Food:	Small fish, insects, carrion.
Voice:	Similar to red-billed gull.
Breeding:	November-December. Two greyish eggs with brown markings.
General:	A scavanger of farm and coastline. Fully protected.

BLACK-FRONTED TERN (Tara) (Whiskered Tern)
Chlidonias albostriatus

See Inside Cover

Size:	30cm.
Status:	Common.
Range:	South Island mainly, migrating to winter in North Island or Stewart Island.
Habitat:	Seashore and river beds.
Description:	Overall grey plumage with bright orange bill and red legs. Crown of head and nape are black with white stripe below eye.
Food:	Flying and water insects.
Voice:	Sharp noted staccato cries.
Breeding:	October-January. One to three stone coloured eggs, dotted brown to grey.
General:	Also known as whiskered tern. Breeds only on South Island river beds east of the Southern Alps. Fully protected.

WHITE-FRONTED TERN (Tara)
Sterna striata

See Inside Cover

Size:	42cm.
Status:	Common.
Range:	Throughout main islands, off-shore islands and some outlying islands. Young birds often migrate to breed in Australia.
Habitat:	Coastal areas and river mouths.
Description:	Head and bill black. White band over bill. Back and tail are ash grey. Legs reddish brown.
Food:	Dives for small fish.
Voice:	Constant low twittering, also harsh whistling note.
Breeding:	October-December. One or two variegated eggs.
General:	Also known as the sea swallow on account of its forked tail. Fully protected.

FURTHER READING	*Annotated Checklist of the Birds of New Zealand* — Ornithological Society of New Zealand. *Common Birds of New Zealand, Vols. 1 & 2* — Marshall/Kinsky/Robertson. *A Field Guide to the Birds of New Zealand* — Falla/Sibson/Turbott. *New Zealand Birds* — Oliver. *New Zealand Birds* — Soper.

Printed in Hong Kong by G. L. Graphic & Printing Limited